Table of Contents

Introduction 3
   Sugar 3
   Sugar Free Diet 5
   Tips For Cutting Out Sugar 8
   Foods To Eat 14
   Foods To Avoid 16
   Reasons Why Sugar Is Bad For You 16
   Other Health Risks 24
   Health Benefits 25
Sugar Free Diet Plan 27
   Breakfast 27
   Lunch 27
   Dinner 27
   Dessert 28
Recipes 28
   Grilled Salmon With Roasted Cauliflower 28
   Turkey Burger With Sautéed Veggies 29
   Three Bean Chili 30
   Greek Yogurt Marinated Chicken 32
   BBQ Chicken Wraps 33
   Lavender Infused Cutlets 34
   Classic Meatballs 35

- Chili Beef 38
- Beef & Lemongrass Skewers 39
- Beef Stoganoff 41
- Crockpot Beef Stew 43
- Verde Salsa Beef 44
- Hungarian Goulash Crockpot 45
- Beef And Vegetable Stir Fry 47
- Dijon Pork Chops 48
- Pork & Kale Rolls 50
- Pumpkin Punch 51
- Almond Meal Cookies 52
- Raspberry Muffins 53
- Fruit Parfait 54
- Roasted Rosemary Almonds 55

Introduction

Many adults eat much more sugar than necessary, so reducing added sugar intake is a healthful idea for most people. Some people may wish to take it a step further and cut sugar out of their diet entirely. The no-sugar diet has gained popularity as people continue to look for effective ways to live a healthful life or lose weight. For all the health benefits of a no-sugar diet, however, there are also a few things to consider. This book explains practical tips to reduce sugar intake, foods to eat and avoid, risks to be aware of as well as recipes.

Sugar

Put simply, sugar is a crystalline carbohydrate that makes foods taste sweet. There are many different types of sugar, including glucose, fructose, lactose, maltose and sucrose – also known as table sugar. Some of these sugars, such as glucose, fructose and lactose, occur naturally in fruits, vegetables and other foods. But many of the foods we consume contain "added" sugars – sugar that we add to a product ourselves to enhance the flavor or sugar that has been added to a product by a manufacturer. The most common sources of added sugars include soft drinks, cakes, pies, chocolate, fruit drinks and desserts. Just a single can of cola can contain up to 7 tsps. of added sugar, while an average-sized chocolate bar can contain up to 6 tsps. It is added sugars that have been cited as a contributor to many health problems. In December 2014, MNT reported on a study in the journal Open Heart claiming added sugars may increase the risk of high blood pressure, even more so than sodium. And in February 2014, a study led by the Centers for Disease Control and Prevention (CDC) associated high added sugar intake with increased risk of death from cardiovascular disease (CVD). Perhaps most strongly, added sugars have been associated with the significant increase in obesity. In the US, more than a third of adults are obese, while the rate of childhood obesity has more than doubled in children and quadrupled in adolescents over the past 30 years. A 2013 study published in The American Journal of Clinical Nutrition suggested that consumption of sugar-sweetened beverages increases weight gain in both children and adults, while a review paper from the World Health Organization (WHO) notes an increase in the consumption of such beverages correlates with the increase in obesity.

Sugar Free Diet

Many adults eat much more sugar than the authorities recommend. The National Institutes of Health (NIH), for example, estimate that adults in the United States get around 15% of their calories from added sugars alone. This sugar intake does not even include natural sugars, such as those in products such as fruit and milk. Excessive sugar consumption has links to several harmful health conditions, including:

- obesity and metabolic syndrome

- heart disease

- type 2 diabetes

- high blood pressure

- high cholesterol

- chronic inflammation

- nonalcoholic fatty liver disease

- dental plaque and cavities

Reducing the amount of sugar in the diet can help a person reduce their risk of these health conditions. Replacing high sugar foods with healthful options can help a person get all of their essential vitamins and minerals without the added calories. It may also help them lose weight, if necessary.

Is eliminating sugar from our diet healthy?

The array of studies reporting the negative implications of added sugar led to WHO making a proposal to revise their added sugar recommendations in 2014. The organization issued a draft guideline stating they would like to halve their recommended daily free sugar intake from 10% to 5%. "The objective of this guideline is to provide recommendations on the consumption of free sugars to reduce the risk of noncommunicable diseases in adults and children," WHO explained, "with a particular focus on the prevention and control of weight gain and dental caries." In addition, it seems many health experts, nutritionists and even celebrities like Gwyneth have jumped on a "no sugar" bandwagon. But is it even possible to completely eliminate sugar from a diet? And is it safe? Biochemist Leah Fitzsimmons, of the University of Birmingham in the UK, told The Daily Mail: "Cutting all sugar from your diet would be very difficult to achieve. Fruits, vegetables, dairy products and dairy replacements, eggs, alcohol and nuts all contain sugar, which would leave you with little other than meat and fats to eat – definitely not very healthy." Many people turn to artificial sweeteners as a sugar alternative, but according to a study reported by MNT in 2014, these sweeteners may still drive diabetes and obesity. The study, published in the journal Nature, suggests artificial sweeteners – including saccharin, sucralose and aspartame – interfere with gut bacteria, increasing the activity of pathways associated with obesity and diabetes. What is more, they found long-term consumption of artificial sweeteners was associated with increased weight, abdominal obesity, higher fasting blood glucose levels and increased glycosylated hemoglobin levels. "Together with other major shifts that occurred in human nutrition, this increase in artificial sweetener consumption coincides with the dramatic increase in the obesity and diabetes epidemics," the authors note. "Our findings suggest that artificial sweeteners may have directly contributed to enhancing the exact epidemic that they themselves were intended to fight."

Tips For Cutting Out Sugar

Here are simple tips a person can use to help cut sugar from their diet:

Take it slow

One of the most important things to remember when changing the diet is to do so gradually. Going from a diet full of sugar to one without any should be a slow process. It may help to start by eliminating the most obvious sources of sugar. People can easily avoid baked goods such as cakes, muffins, and brownies. Removing candy and sugary beverages is also an excellent place to start. A person can also try reducing the amount of sugar and cream they add to their coffee or tea, working up to using none at all. Building up to a no-sugar diet can help a person retrain the palate, meaning that they are less likely to crave the missing sugar.

Read product labels

Once a person has managed to cut out the most obvious sugar from their diet, they can turn their attention to other products that contain sugar. Reading product labels can help them identify types of sugars to avoid. Sugar has many names and is in many different syrups and concentrates. There are at least 61 different names for sugar on food labels. The most common ones include:

- cane sugar

- brown sugar

- corn syrup or high fructose corn syrup

- evaporated cane juice

- invert sugar

- beet sugar

- barley malt

- coconut sugar

- maple syrup

- agave syrup

- rice syrup

- apple or grape juice concentrate

- honey

- demerara

- sucanat

- panela or piloncillo

- turbinado

- muscovado

People should also be aware that any item on an ingredients list ending "-ose" is also a type of sugar. Examples of these ingredients include:

- sucrose

- glucose

- dextrose

- fructose

- lactose

Sugars hide in many different supermarket foods. Reading the label is a must for people who want to follow a no-sugar diet. Products such as salad dressing and condiments, pasta sauce, breakfast cereals, milk, and granola bars often have sugar in their ingredients list.

Avoid simple carbohydrates

Many no-sugar diets also recommend that people avoid simple carbohydrates. Simple carbs include white flour, white pasta, and white rice. The body quickly breaks down the carbohydrates in these foods into sugar. This process causes a spike in blood sugar levels. A person can usually replace simple carbs with whole grain options.

Avoid artificial sugars

Artificial sugars are a subject of controversy in the diet industry. They are much sweeter than sugar but contain few or no calories. However, eating artificial sugars can trick the body into thinking that it is actually eating sugar. This can intensify a person's sugar cravings, making it more difficult for them to stick to a no-sugar diet. For this reason, a person following a no-sugar diet should avoid artificial sugars such as:

- Splenda

- stevia

- Equal

- NutraSweet

- Sweet'N Low

People can also look for the chemical names of these sweeteners on ingredients lists, especially in anything marketed as low sugar, low calorie, or diet food. Chemical names include:

- aspartame

- sucralose

- saccharin

- acesulfame K or acesulfame potassium

- neotame

Do not drink sugar

Sugar may be easy to avoid in processed foods. However, sugar sweetened drinks are among the most significant sources of added sugars in the diet. These include soda, specialty coffee, sweetened teas, and fruit juices. Replacing these drinks with unsweetened herbal tea, coffee without sugar, sparkling mineral water, or just water can help a person stay hydrated without increasing their sugar intake.

Focus on whole foods

A person following a no-sugar diet should also aim to eat whole foods. Processed foods are more likely to contain refined ingredients or added sugars. Diets that focus on whole and complete foods include the following options:

- vegetables

- fruits

- lean meats, poultry, or tofu

- fish

- whole, unprocessed grains, and legumes

- nuts and seeds

Some people might choose to keep a small amount of dairy in their diet, such as plain yogurt, simple cheeses, and milk.

Plan meals

Sticking to a diet with no plan is difficult. When a person feels hungry, they may be more likely to reach for a sugary snack if they do not have nutritious meals and healthful alternatives to hand. Many people take a day to do both their shopping and meal preparation for the entire week.

With healthful food ready to go, they have less temptation to reach for a candy bar or soda.

Spice it up

The palate often misses sugar because it has no other flavors to replace it. However, people can easily add many sweet tasting herbs and spices to foods and drinks to replace sugar. Common replacements include cinnamon, nutmeg, cardamom, and vanilla. These can be a flavorsome addition to coffee, oatmeal, or yogurt.

Foods To Eat

Below are list of food to eat on a sugar free diet:

• Animal proteins (beef, chicken, turkey, pork, fish, etc.)

• Unrefined oils (avocado, coconut, olive, etc.)

• Butter, ghee, cheese

• Avocado

• Eggplant

• Green beans

• Kelp noodles

- Zucchini noodles
- Mushrooms
- Spinach
- Watercress
- Radish
- Kale
- Celery
- Broccoli
- Bell pepper
- Cucumber
- Asparagus
- Tomato
- Mustard
- Salsa
- Coffee
- Tea

- Watermelon

- Lemons/limes

- Whole milk

- Berries

Foods To Avoid

Foods containing added sugar. Sweets such as candy, pastries, sweetened drinks (sodas and high-sugar energy and sports drinks), sweetened foods (such as yogurt with fruit on the bottom).

Reasons Why Sugar Is Bad For You

Can Cause Weight Gain

Rates of obesity are rising worldwide and added sugar, especially from sugar-sweetened beverages, is thought to be one of the main culprits. Sugar-sweetened drinks like sodas, juices and sweet teas are loaded with fructose, a type of simple sugar. Consuming fructose increases your hunger and desire for food more than glucose, the main type of sugar found in starchy foods. Additionally, excessive fructose consumption may cause resistance to leptin, an important hormone that regulates hunger and tells your body to stop eating. In other words, sugary beverages don't curb your hunger, making it easy to quickly consume a high number of liquid calories. This can lead to weight gain. Research has consistently shown that people who drink sugary beverages, such as soda and juice, weigh more than people who don't. Also, drinking a lot of sugar-sweetened beverages is linked to an increased amount of visceral fat, a kind of deep belly fat associated with conditions like diabetes and heart disease.

May Increase Your Risk of Heart Disease

High-sugar diets have been associated with an increased risk of many diseases, including heart disease, the number one cause of death worldwide. Evidence suggests that high-sugar diets can lead to obesity, inflammation and high triglyceride, blood sugar and blood pressure levels — all risk factors for heart disease. Additionally, consuming too much sugar, especially from sugar-sweetened drinks, has been linked to atherosclerosis, a disease characterized by fatty, artery-clogging deposits. A study in over 30,000 people found that those who consumed 17–21% of calories from added sugar had a 38% greater risk of dying from heart disease, compared to those consuming only 8% of calories from added sugar. Just one 16-ounce (473-ml) can of soda contains 52 grams of sugar, which equates to more than 10% of your daily calorie consumption, based on a 2,000-calorie diet.

Has Been Linked to Acne

A diet high in refined carbs, including sugary foods and drinks, has been associated with a higher risk of developing acne. Foods with a high glycemic index, such as processed sweets, raise your blood sugar more rapidly than foods with a lower glycemic index. Sugary foods quickly spike blood sugar and insulin levels, causing increased androgen secretion, oil production and inflammation, all of which play a role in acne development. Studies have shown that low-glycemic diets are associated with a reduced acne risk, while high-glycemic diets are linked to a greater risk. For example, a study in 2,300 teens demonstrated that those who frequently consumed added sugar had a 30% greater risk of developing acne. Also, many population studies have shown that rural communities that consume traditional, non-processed foods have almost non-existent rates of acne, compared to more urban, high-income areas. These findings coincide with the theory that diets high in processed, sugar-laden foods contribute to the development of acne.

Increases Your Risk of Type 2 Diabetes

The worldwide prevalence of diabetes has more than doubled over the past 30 years. Though there are many reasons for this, there is a clear link between excessive sugar consumption and diabetes risk. Obesity, which is often caused by consuming too much sugar, is considered the strongest risk factor for diabetes. What's more, prolonged high-sugar consumption drives resistance to insulin, a hormone produced by the pancreas that regulates blood sugar levels. Insulin resistance causes blood sugar levels to rise and strongly increases your risk of diabetes. A population study comprising over 175 countries found that the risk of developing diabetes grew by 1.1% for every 150 calories of sugar, or about one can of soda, consumed per day. Other studies have also shown that people who drink sugar-sweetened beverages, including fruit juice, are more likely to develop diabetes.

May Increase Your Risk of Cancer

Eating excessive amounts of sugar may increase your risk of developing certain cancers. First, a diet rich in sugary foods and beverages can lead to obesity, which significantly raises your risk of cancer. Furthermore, diets high in sugar increase inflammation in your body and may cause insulin resistance, both of which increase cancer risk. A study in over 430,000 people found that added sugar consumption was positively associated with an increased risk of esophageal cancer, pleural cancer and cancer of the small intestine. Another study showed that women who consumed sweet buns and cookies more than three times per week were 1.42 times more likely to develop endometrial cancer than women who consumed these foods less than 0.5 times per week. Research on the link between added sugar intake and cancer is ongoing, and more studies are needed to fully understand this complex relationship.

May Increase Your Risk of Depression

While a healthy diet can help improve your mood, a diet high in added sugar and processed foods may increase your chances of developing depression. Consuming a lot of processed foods, including high-sugar products such as cakes and sugary drinks, has been associated with a higher risk of depression. Researchers believe that blood sugar swings, neurotransmitter dysregulation and inflammation may all be reasons for sugar's detrimental impact on mental health. A study following 8,000 people for 22 years showed that men who consumed 67 grams or more of sugar per day were 23% more likely to develop depression than men who ate less than 40 grams per day. Another study in over 69,000 women demonstrated that those with the highest intakes of added sugars had a significantly greater risk of depression, compared to those with the lowest intakes.

May Accelerate the Skin Aging Process

Wrinkles are a natural sign of aging. They appear eventually, regardless of your health. However, poor food choices can worsen wrinkles and speed the skin aging process. Advanced glycation end products (AGEs) are compounds formed by reactions between sugar and protein in your body. They are suspected to play a key role in skin aging. Consuming a diet high in refined carbs and sugar leads to the production of AGEs, which may cause your skin to age prematurely. AGEs damage collagen and elastin, which are proteins that help the skin stretch and keep its youthful appearance. When collagen and elastin become damaged, the skin loses its firmness and begins to sag. In one study, women who consumed more carbs, including added sugars, had a more wrinkled appearance than women on a high-protein, lower-carb diet. The researchers concluded that a lower intake of carbs was associated with better skin-aging appearance.

Can Increase Cellular Aging

Telomeres are structures found at the end of chromosomes, which are molecules that hold part or all of your genetic information. Telomeres act as protective caps, preventing chromosomes from deteriorating or fusing together. As you grow older, telomeres naturally shorten, which causes cells to age and malfunction. Although the shortening of telomeres is a normal part of aging, unhealthy lifestyle choices can speed up the process. Consuming high amounts of sugar has been shown to accelerate telomere shortening, which increases cellular aging. A study in 5,309 adults showed that regularly drinking sugar-sweetened beverages was associated with shorter telomere length and premature cellular aging. In fact, each daily 20-ounce (591-ml) serving of sugar-sweetened soda equated to 4.6 additional years of aging, independent of other variables.

Drains Your Energy

Foods high in added sugar quickly spike blood sugar and insulin levels, leading to increased energy. However, this rise in energy levels is fleeting. Products that are loaded with sugar but lacking in protein, fiber or fat lead to a brief energy boost that's quickly followed by a sharp drop in blood sugar, often referred to as a crash. Having constant blood sugar swings can lead to major fluctuations in energy levels. To avoid this energy-draining cycle, choose carb sources that are low in added sugar and rich in fiber. Pairing carbs with protein or fat is another great way to keep your blood sugar and energy levels stable. For example, eating an apple along with a small handful of almonds is an excellent snack for prolonged, consistent energy levels.

Can Lead to Fatty Liver

A high intake of fructose has been consistently linked to an increased risk of fatty liver. Unlike glucose and other types of sugar, which are taken up by many cells throughout the body, fructose is almost exclusively broken down by the liver. In the liver, fructose is converted into energy or stored as glycogen. However, the liver can only store so much glycogen before excess amounts are turned into fat. Large amounts of added sugar in the form of fructose overload your liver, leading to non-alcoholic fatty liver disease (NAFLD), a condition characterized by excessive fat buildup in the liver. A study in over 5,900 adults showed that people who drank sugar-sweetened beverages daily had a 56% higher risk of developing NAFLD, compared to people who did not.

Other Health Risks

Aside from the risks listed above, sugar can harm your body in countless other ways. Research shows that too much added sugar can:

• Increase kidney disease risk: Having consistently high blood sugar levels can cause damage to the delicate blood vessels in your kidneys. This can lead to an increased risk of kidney disease.

• Negatively impact dental health: Eating too much sugar can cause cavities. Bacteria in your mouth feed on sugar and release acid byproducts, which cause tooth demineralization.

• Increase the risk of developing gout: Gout is an inflammatory condition characterized by pain in the joints. Added sugars raise uric acid levels in the blood, increasing the risk of developing or worsening gout.

• Accelerate cognitive decline: High-sugar diets can lead to impaired memory and have been linked to an increased risk of dementia.

Research on the impact of added sugar on health is ongoing, and new discoveries are constantly being made.

Health Benefits

Eliminating added sugars and maintaining a diet rich in whole foods has many benefits for the body. Specifically, reducing sugar intake and eating a healthful diet may help people:

• lose weight and prevent obesity, according to one 2019 article in the journal Medical Clinics of North America

• have clearer skin and reduce the risk of skin cancer, according to a 2014 review in The Journal of Clinical and Aesthetic Dermatology

• prevent mood shifts, as a 2017 study linked a high sugar diet with changing mood states

• reduce inflammation, according to one 2018 review of studies

• reduce the risk of type 2 diabetes, as sugar can increase the risk of obesity, which can lead to type 2 diabetes

Risks And Considerations

Before adopting a no-sugar diet, a person should consider whether or not they also want to eliminate natural sugars. Natural sugars occur in fruit and some dairy products. Although the proponents of some no-sugar diet plans say that a person should eliminate fruit, this may not be the most healthful choice. Fruit can provide several essential nutrients, including fiber, antioxidants, and other healthful compounds that help protect the body from disease. Including whole fruits in a no-sugar diet can still be healthful. However, if a person chooses to eat dried fruit, they should do so in moderation and look for varieties without added sugar. Eliminating sugar from the diet is not a complete solution for weight loss. It is part of a lifestyle change that should also involve regular exercise and a nutritious diet. Anyone looking to start following a no-sugar diet should speak to a doctor, dietitian, or nutritionist, especially if they have any underlying health conditions.

Sugar Free Diet Plan
Breakfast
- 2 eggs, any style

- 1/2 avocado

- 1 cup zucchini, sautéed with olive oil

Snack

- 8 walnut halves

Lunch
- 3 oz. grilled chicken (breast or thighs)

- 1 cup of steamed cauliflower with 1 oz. melted cheese

- 1 cup steamed green beans

Dinner
- 3 oz. wild-caught salmon, baked

- 1 cup asparagus and 1 cup mushrooms, sauteed in 2 tbsp ghee butter

Dessert
- 8g 100% dark chocolate shavings with 2 tbsp coconut whipped cream

Recipes

Grilled Salmon With Roasted Cauliflower

Ingredients

- 5 oz. wild salmon filet
- 2 tsp. extra virgin, cold-pressed olive oil
- 1/2 tsp. pepper
- 2 cups cauliflower
- 1/4 tsp. garlic powder
- 1/4 tsp. sea salt

Directions:

- Preheat oven to 425°Fahrenheit.

- Pat salmon fillet dry with a paper towel, and rub with 1 teaspoon olive oil and pepper to taste. Place onto a nonstick baking sheet skin side down.

- On a separate baking sheet, break cauliflower into small florets and lay evenly in a single layer. Drizzle with 1 teaspoon olive oil and sprinkle generously with remaining pepper, garlic, and sea salt.

- Place both trays in the oven and allow to roast for about 12-15 minutes, or until the salmon flakes easily with a fork and the cauliflower is roasted and slightly browned.

Turkey Burger With Sautéed Veggies
Ingredients:

- 1 tbsp. extra virgin, cold-pressed olive oil

- 1/3 cup red onion, thinly sliced

- 1/2 cup bell pepper, thinly sliced

- 4 oz. frozen turkey burger, thawed

- 2 cups kale, chopped

- 1 cup cherry tomatoes, halved

- 1/4 tsp. sea salt

- 1/2 tsp. pepper

Directions:

- Drizzle olive oil into a nonstick pan over medium heat.

- Add onion and peppers and cook until tender and aromatic, about 5 minutes.

- While veggies are cooking, place the turkey burger in a clean, small pan over medium heat. Cook until done, flipping halfway through, for about 5-7 minutes, or according to directions.

- To the veggies, add kale and tomatoes, and cook until kale is wilted and soft, about 3 minutes. Season veggies with sea salt and pepper to taste.

- Transfer cooked turkey burger to plate, top with sautéed veggie mixture, and enjoy!

Three Bean Chili
Ingredients

- 2 tsp. olive oil

- 1 onion, chopped

- 1 red bell pepper, chopped

- 1 yellow bell pepper, chopped

- 2 tsp. cumin

- 2 tsp. chili powder

- 1 15-oz. can kidney beans, drained

- 1 15-oz. can garbanzo beans, drained

- 1 15-oz. can black beans, drained

- 1 1/2 cups frozen yellow corn, defrosted

- 2 15-oz. cans diced tomatoes (with liquid)

- salt and pepper to taste

Directions:

- Heat olive oil in a large sauce pan over medium heat.

- To the pan, add onion, bell peppers, cumin, and chili powder.

- Cook until vegetables are tender, stirring occasionally.

- Add kidney beans, garbanzo beans, black beans, corn, and diced tomatoes.

- Add salt and pepper to taste.

- Reduce to medium-low heat, and allow to simmer for 45 minutes. Serve warm.

Greek Yogurt Marinated Chicken

Ingredients

- 1 cup low-fat Greek yogurt
- 1 tbsp. extra virgin, cold-pressed olive oil
- 1 tsp. chili powder
- 1 garlic clove, minced
- 1/4 tsp. sea salt
- 1/4 tsp. pepper
- 2 pounds chicken breast

Directions:

- Whisk the yogurt, olive oil, chili powder, garlic, salt, and pepper in a bowl.

- Place chicken in a container and pour marinade over the breasts. Cover and let sit in the refrigerator overnight.

- Preheat grill.

- Remove chicken from marinade and grill over medium heat until chicken is cooked through.

BBQ Chicken Wraps
Ingredients

- ½ cup pureed natural apricots, or honey
- ¼ cup apple cider vinegar
- 1 tsp paprika
- 4 skinless chicken thigh or breast fillets
- 8 slices bacon rashers

Directions:

- Whisk apricot puree or honey, vinegar and smoked paprika together in a saucepan over med-high heat. Simmer for approx. 8 minutes or until thickened.
- Preheat grill to med-high or use a BBQ
- Slice bacon into thirds. Chop chicken into cubes
- Placing an individual cube of chicken onto each bacon slice; wrap it around chicken and place onto skewer. Repeat with 3-4 pieces on each skewer.
- Brush all sides of bacon-wrapped chicken skewers with honey glaze.

- Cook on hot grill or BBQ turning every 2-3 minutes. Brush with more glaze and cook for about 8-10 minutes.

*Serve with salad greens & parsley. BBQ eggplant & zucchini or steamed veggies go very nicely too!

Lavender Infused Cutlets
You can soak the cutlets in the marinade first if you wish.

Ingredients:

- 8 lamb cutlets, beef works too

- 1 onion, finely chopped

- 3 Tbsp finely chopped fresh lavender

- 2 Tbsp olive oil

- 1 Tbsp red wine or white vinegar (red wine and white vinegar has nil g of sugar, balsamic 15g, and cider 0.4g of sugar per 100g)

- 1 Tbsp lemon juice

- raw salt and ground black pepper to taste

Directions:

- Place the cutlets in a large bowl, mix in the onion.

- Add the lavender.

- In a small bowl beat together the olive oil, vinegar and lemon juice. Pour over the cutlets. Add the seasonings.

- Coat the meat.

- Barbecue the meat, or grill on the stove top basting with the marinade until golden brown, turning as you go. Delicious served with a coleslaw, garden salad or just as finger food.

Classic Meatballs

Ingredients: for the meatballs

- 1 pound or about 500gm lean beef mince

- 1 pound or about 500gm lean pork mince

- 1 1/2 Tbsp chopped fresh parsley

- 1 Tbs chopped fresh oregano or marjoram

- 1 tsp fresh or dried basil

- 2 garlic cloves, crushed and chopped

- 4 small fresh button mushrooms

- 1 egg

- 1 Tbsp olive oil
- black pepper
- raw salt

Ingredients: for the Sauce

- 1 large finely chopped onion
- 150ml dry red wine (about 1g of sugar per 100g)
- 2 cups of canned tomatoes (2.4g of sugar per 100g)
- 1 Tbsp full cream
- 1/2 cup water
- 1 tsp salt
- pinch of ground black pepper
- 1 tsp ground fresh chili (optional)
- 1 tsp fresh or dried oregano
- fresh basil or chives to garnish

Directions: for meatballs

- Heat the skillet of frying pan to medium and add oil and onion, frying for 2-3 minutes or until slightly golden.

- Place all the ingredients including the onion into a large bowl and mix thoroughly using your hands. Make sure to "knead" the mixture for a few minutes to bind everything together properly.

- Wet your hands, roll the meat mixture into small balls the size of a golf ball.

- Heat the same frying pan to medium high, add some oil and place meatballs into pan. Cook for about 5 -6 minutes on "each side" until done.

Directions: for sauce

- Heat same pan to medium - add some extra oil to the pan and saute onion for about 4 minutes (in the same frying pan)

- De-glaze the pan with the red wine and bring to a simmer. Add the tomatoes, cream, chili, oregano, water, salt and pepper and bring to the simmer again.

- Serve with cocktail sticks or skewers accompanied with homemade tomato ketchup.

Chili Beef

Chili Beef is one of those simple traditional favorites loved by kids and adults! You can add some extra healthy veggies or even vegetable puree for those fussy eaters. Red kidney beans only have 0.3g of sugar, but they have 23g of carbs, so add some if you like.

Ingredients:

- 2 Tbsp olive oil

- 1 diced onion

- 6 stalks of celery (diced)

- 4 garlic cloves (minced)

- 3 1/2 pounds (about 1.3kg) ground beef

- 4 tsp cumin

- 4 tsp chilli powder

- 4 tsp oregano

- 2 Tbsp BBQ seasoning

- 2 x 8 oz cans of diced tomatoes

- 1 small can tomato paste or puree

- green chillies to taste

- 4 tsp sea salt

Directions:

- Using a large pot; fry onions, celery and garlic in oil over med-high heat. Cook for about 4 minutes adding beef and spices and seasonings. Cook for further 5 minutes; stirring constantly.

- Add tomatoes, paste or puree, chillies and salt. Simmer for about 1 hour.

- Add a small bunch of chopped parsley at the end of cooking if desired.

*Wonderful as a stand by freezer dinner of lunch!

Beef & Lemongrass Skewers

This is very flexible with the meat used and the herbs - I like using rosemary too if it's in the garden. Cilantro/ coriander can be substituted or mixed with rosemary, or even removed all together.

Ingredients:

- 1 pound, about 500 g lean tenderloin beef, cut into small cubes (about 1 1/2 inches)
- 2 cloves garlic, finely chopped
- 4 lemongrass stalks
- 2 Tbsp natural fish sauce (can use anchovies)
- 2 Tbsp sesame oil (nil g of sugar or carbs)
- 2 Tbsp natural maple syrup or Stevia equivalent (maple syrup has 68g of sugar per 100g)
- 1 1/2 tsp ground five spice powder
- 1 small bunch of coriander/cilantro, finely chopped

*Soak wooden skewers in water for 1 hour beforehand to stop burning.

Directions:

- Prepare the lemongrass by cutting away the top 2 thirds and outer leaves, just using the tender part. Chop finely, or blend.
- Mix together the garlic, lemongrass, fish sauce, sesame oil, maple syrup, 5 spice and coriander in a bowl.

- Cut beef into cubes and marinate in the lemongrass mix for at least 20 mins.

- Thread desired amount onto skewers evenly and fry in oil on stove top or BBQ grill.

*Accompany with favorite dip, salad or salsa. You can either remove or leave on the skewers.

Beef Stoganoff

This can be cooked on the stove top or slow cooked in the crockpot. Mushrooms are high in nutrition.

Ingredients:

- 3 pounds or about 1360g, any stewing meat, cubed

- 6 oz or about 170g mushrooms, sliced (about 2g of sugar per 100g and about 4g of carbs)

- 2 cups homemade beef stock (although bought only has around 1.2g of sugar, but not as nutritious)

- ½ cup low carb flour for thickening

- 1 onion, diced

- 1 tsp Tabasco sauce (nil g sugar)

- 1 Tbsp Homemade Tomato Sauce
- 1 tsp salt
- ¼ tsp garlic flakes (fresh will work)
- ¼ tsp black pepper
- ½ cup sour cream, or similar (2.9g of sugar per 100g and 2.9g of carbs)

Directions:

- Brown the meat and onion in a little oil on the stove top first.
- Place the meat, onion salt & pepper in a crock pot.
- In a small bowl combine the beef stock, Tabasco, sauce and garlic. Pour this sauce over the meat. Cook for 8 hours on low or 4 hours on high.
- Half an hour before serving whisk together the flour and a little of the juice from the crock pot. Pour the sauce back into the crock pot and mix it in briskly. Mix in the mushrooms, and cook on high for 30 minutes.
- Stir in the cream just before serving.

*Serve with rice or vegetables.

Crockpot Beef Stew

Ingredients:

- 1 Tbsp olive oil

- 1 pound or about 500g lean finely diced or minced beef

- 1 medium brown onion, chopped

- 1 green of red bell pepper, chopped

- 2 cups fresh mixed vegetables such as broccoli, kale, green beans, carrots etc.

- 2 large tins of tomatoes, or about half a dozen fresh home grown.

- 2 cups beef stock and/or water

- Salt, garlic flakes (or fresh) and ground black pepper to taste

Directions:

- Brown minced beef and onion in frypan. Add bell pepper and cook for a few minutes.

- Transfer to large heavy saucepan or the crockpot.

- Add remaining ingredients; cover and cook for 4 hours on low setting or simmer on the stove top for about an hour.

Verde Salsa Beef
Ingredients:

- 1 sliced tomato (2.6g of sugar per 100g and 3.9g of carbs)

- ½ cup parsley leaves

- ½ cup basil leaves

- 3 cloves garlic

- 2 Tbsp capers (drained)

- 1 anchovy fillet, cut into pieces (nil sugar, nil carbs)

- 1 cup olive oil

- 2 Tbsp fresh lime juice

- salt to taste

- 1 - 2 tsp of black peppercorns (3 color blend is good too)

- 750g (about 25oz) lean sirloin/ fillet steak or similar piece of roasting beef

*Sprinkle with fresh rosemary to garnish

Directions:

- Purée parsley, basil, garlic, capers, tomato and anchovy fillet in blender; slowly add olive oil until combined. Add lime juice, salt and pepper blending till well combined and smooth. Adjust seasonings to taste and set sauce aside.

- Season and grill or pan fry steak to your particular preference.

- When cooked; slice thinly and drizzle with salsa verde. Garnish with some rosemary sprigs or herbs of your choice.

Hungarian Goulash Crockpot

Ingredients:

- 3 1/2 pounds beef, cut into largish cubes

- raw salt and ground black pepper to taste

- 1 Tbsp low carb flour to thicken stew

- 1 Tbsp Hungarian paprika

- 1/4 tsp caraway seeds

- 2 Tbsp coconut oil

- 1 eggplant cut into small pieces or grated (optional. carrot works too)

- 1 large onion, chopped finely

- 3 cloves chopped garlic

- 1 bay leaf

- 1 1/2 red bell peppers cut into chunks

- 1 medium can diced tomatoes

- 1/2 - 1 cup of beef stock if you like more of a soup style (optional)

*A few potatoes can be added to this recipe 3/4 of the way through cooking if desired

Directions:

- Season the beef with salt, pepper and sprinkle with flour.

- Heat a large skillet or stock pot to medium high. Brown the meat in half the coconut oil then remove from pan.

- In same pan add rest of oil and add the onion and garlic, stirring while sauteing for about 3 minutes. Add paprika and caraway seeds for just a minute and stir through, taking care not to burn. This will make the dish bitter.

- De-glaze the pan with the stock or tomatoes and now add all the remaining ingredients. Cook for about 10 minutes, then transfer to your slow cooker. Usually takes about 6 hours on low. You can add some vegetables like kale or spinach if you wish. If desired this dish can be cooked on the stove top.

Beef And Vegetable Stir Fry

I always use onions or spring onions in this stir fry, although the other veggies are inter changeable.

Ingredients:

- 1 pound or about 16oz of lean beef, pork or chicken, sliced into strips

- 1 Tbsp olive oil for cooking

- 5 cups of assorted bite sized pieces of onion, broccoli, bell capsicum pepper, spring

- onion, mushrooms, bok choy, carrot. (the vegetables that work are up to you. Use what you have. I change it up with cauliflower, Chinese cabbage, sprouts etc.)

- 2 cloves chopped garlic (optional)

- 3 tsp curry paste

- 1/2 tsp chili (optional - dried flakes or fresh)

- 2 - 3 Tbsp full cream (optional)

- 1 tsp raw salt, or to taste

Directions:

- Heat wok or frying pan to medium high. Add 1/2 the oil and stir fry the vegetables for about 5 minutes tossing constantly.

- Add the curry paste, keep stirring for another few minutes till flavors are released. Remove to a dish.

- Heat wok to high and add remainder oil to the wok and put in the beef strips, garlic and chili. Cook for a further 3 minutes until almost done, then tip all the vegetables back in along with the coconut milk, salt and sesame seeds.

- Toss all together for a few minutes more. Serve with fresh herbs, mashed cauliflower or flat bread.

Dijon Pork Chops
Ingredients:

- 4 lean pork chops

- Salt and pepper to taste

- ½ cup Dijon mustard (mustard(s) have about 0.9g of sugar per 100g and about 5g of carbs)

- 1 tsp mustard powder

- 1 tsp dried thyme

- 1 tsp garlic (minced)

- 1 Tbsp olive oil

Directions:

- Preheat oven to 425°F.

- Season pork chops with salt & pepper.

- Combine mustard, mustard powder, thyme & garlic in a small bowl. Mix well. Spread evenly over both sides of pork chops.

- Heat oil in a large frypan over medium-high, add chops and brown for about 2 minutes per side.

- Transfer chops to baking dish and cook in oven for another 5-8 minutes or until cooked through.

- Serve over sautéed baby spinach and/or a scrumptious fresh green salad.

Pork & Kale Rolls
Ingredients:

- 1 pound or about 500g pork tenderloin (any meat leftovers works well)

- 150g kale leaves (cabbage or spinach works well too)

- 2 garlic cloves

- spices for meat: thyme, chilli or any other spices you like

- olive oil

Directions:

- Cut the pork in slices, soften it with a meat mallet. Sprinkle the meat slices generously with a mix of chopped garlic and spices.

- Blanche the kale leaves, then dry them and put them atop of the pork.

- Create rolls out of them. Heat up some oil in a frying pan.

- Once it is hot, fry the rolls on medium to high heat. These can be steamed if desired instead.

Pumpkin Punch

Pumpkin and banana are quite high in sugars, but this recipe has been added for its nutritional value. Eat in moderation or for a special treat. Another option is to use 1 cup of berries instead of banana. Mix up your own recipes with whatever you have on hand. Get creative, this is how yummy recipes are born!

Ingredients:

- 1/2 cup of pumpkin puree (pumpkin has 2.8g of sugar per 100g and 6g of carbs)

- 1 tsp mixed spice (or cinnamon)

- 1/2 tsp vanilla extract

- 3/4 cup unsweetened almond milk

- 1 chilled or frozen banana or berries (banana is high at 12g of sugar per 100g and 23g carbs)

- 6-7 ice cubes

- honey to taste (I use about 2 tsp)

Directions:

- Blender until smooth. Garnish with mint and some nutmeg if desired.

Almond Meal Cookies

Ingredients:

- 1 Tbsp coconut flour

- 3/4 cup almond meal

- 1 large egg

- 1 Tbsp raw honey, maple syrup or Stevia equivalent

- 1/2 tsp vanilla extract

- 1/3 tsp baking soda

- 4 Tbs coconut or olive oil

- 2 Tbs crushed unsalted cashew nuts (I also use almonds, walnuts or macadamia nuts)

Directions:

- Preheat oven to a moderate 350F.

- Spray baking tray or sheet with coconut oil spray or line with baking paper.

- In a medium sized mixer bowl, mix together the almond meal, coconut flour, coconut and baking soda. Add the wet ingredients and mix well.

- Use a spoon or a small scoop and place smallish "ping pong ball sized" drops of mix onto the tray. With the back of a fork gently press down to flatten.

- Place in the moderate oven and bake for about 8-10 minutes. Let the cookies cool for at least 5 minutes so they can set or firm up.

Raspberry Muffins
Ingredients:

- 1 cup almond or low carb flour

- 1 tsp baking powder

- pinch of salt

- 1 cup softened natural butter, or almond butter

- 1 cup fresh raspberries, or blackberries

- ½ cup olive oil

- ¼ cup raw honey, maple syrup or Stevia equivalent

- 3 eggs, whisked

- ¼ cup slivered or flaked almonds

Directions:

- Preheat oven to 350°F

- In a medium - large size bowl mix together all dry ingredients: almond flour, baking powder and salt.

- In another bowl combine butter, honey, oil and eggs mixing well.

- Gently combine the wet ingredients and raspberries into the dry.

- Scoop the batter in slightly greased muffin cups (or use paper muffin liners). Cover each muffin with sliced almonds as decoration.

- Bake for 15-20 minutes.

Fruit Parfait

Oats is low in sugar and low in GI making it good for a satisfying breakfast. It is high in carbs but fiber too. So, eat in moderation.

Ingredients:

- ¾ cup fruit of your choice (apricot and cranberries are good)

- ½ cup oatmeal (oats have 0.3g of sugar per 100g and 66g of carbs)

- ½ cup skim ricotta

- ½ tsp flavoring (such as almond, vanilla or lemon)

- dash of cinnamon

- dash of nutmeg

Directions:

- Preheat the oven to 350°F (180°C). Spread the oats on a baking sheet. Bake for 10 minutes until lightly brown. Mix in cinnamon and nutmeg. Let the oats cool.

- Meanwhile mix ricotta with your favorite flavoring and cut the fruit in small bite-size pieces.

- Once the oats have cooled, alternate layers of oats, ricotta and fruit in a serving bowl. Enjoy!

Roasted Rosemary Almonds

Try any assortment of nuts and seeds you like. Almonds have 4.6g of sugar per 100g and 18g of carbs.

Ingredients:

- 1 1/2 cups raw almonds with skin on (can use other nuts like hazelnuts, cashews and macadamias)
- 1 Tbsp butter
- 1 Tbsp fresh rosemary, minced (use the whole sprig)
- 1 clove of garlic, minced
- salt and ground black pepper to taste
- 2 tsp Worcestershire or Tabasco sauce

Directions:

- Preheat oven to 350° F
- In a large nonstick skillet pan heated to medium, fry the rosemary and garlic in the butter or oil for 10 seconds until the aromas are released.
- Add the almonds and seasoning, stirring quickly for about 1 min, making sure the almonds are coated well with the spice mix. If you want to use seeds, add them last.
- Pour over the source again mixing quickly for about 1 min.

- Place the nuts onto a baking tray and bake until the nut are toasted, about 5 to 10 mins.

*Serve immediately, or cool and place in an airtight container in the refrigerator for up to 2 days.

Printed in Great Britain
by Amazon